dr Anne Good Health At Hand

QUICK START!

Also by Anne Seifert:

His, Mine, & Ours:
A guide to keeping marriage from ruining a perfectly good relationship.
Macmillan, 1979 ISBN:0026090309

The Intelligent Woman's Diet:
The practical way to keep trim, relax, and stay well the rest of your life.
Varnes Publishers, 1982 ISBN:0943584019

Contributor, Voices of Survival:
In the nuclear age, by Dennis Paulson, Capra Press, 1986

Dr. Anne's Magic-Hand Eating Plan:
Good health, happiness and weight control.
Varnes Publishers, 2004 ISBN:9780943584034

Contributor, To Be With God:
Despite limitations of the brain, by Edward A. Siegel, M.D.
CreateSpace, 2010

Dr.Anne Good Health at Hand (Expanded Edition)
Your own lifelong way to eat, exercise and meditate
Varnes Publishers, 2022 ISBN:9780943584065

Anne Seifert books available through online & other bookstores.

dr.Anne Good Health At Hand

Your own lifelong way to eat, exercise and meditate

By Anne Seifert, M.P.H. Ph.D.

Varnes Publishers
Seal Beach, California

Varnes Publishers
Seal Beach, CA
Varnespubs@email.com

Library of Congress Cataloguing in Publication Data

Seifert, Anne M.
Dr. Anne Good Health At Hand: Your own lifelong way to eat, exercise and meditate
ISBN:978-0-943584-04-1
1. Health & Fitness 2. Diet & Nutrition 3. Weight loss

Library of Congress Control Number: 2020939565

First Edition
Second Printing August 2023
Printed in United States of America

Illustration and Image Credits

Back cover. sitting Buddha (modified): designed by Freepik.com *<a href="https://www.freepik.com/free-photos-vectors/background">Background vector created by freepik - www.freepik.com</a>*

Page 5. Photo enhanced by Stan Johnson

Page 8. Photo c. Fred Hoyt

Page 14. Foods— Apple emoji

Page 35, 37. Silhouettes (modified) Man and woman, Apple people shapes

Page 61. Two hands (modified): Apple unicode emoji

Disclaimer:

The purpose of this book is to educate the reader about well-balanced nutrition and to provide a lifelong food-based portion-control program for good health and weight control. Individual results may vary. There is no guarantee as to how much weight will be lost following this program. The instruction given will for most people improve their general nutrition, health, and foster gradual safe weight loss.
It is offered with the understanding that each person is different, and it is the responsibility of the individual to check first with a health professional if there is any concern that the advice included herein might not apply for a specific situation or medical condition. Every effort has been made to make this a flexible and adaptable program. Readers are urged to tailor this information-- how to eat, exercise and meditate-- to meet their individual needs.
Simply stated, know your own body and use your common sense when changing lifestyle habits.

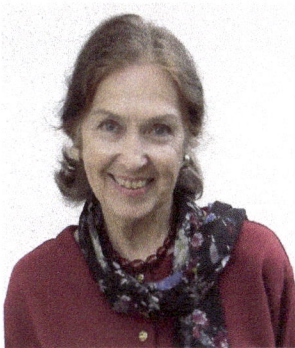

About the Author

Background Summary: Ph.D. and M.P.H. from U.C. Berkeley in epidemiology; M.A. from Smith College in Experimental Psychology; B.A. Psychology from Hofstra University; Harvard University researcher, Department of Nutrition; Columbia University College of Physicians & Surgeons. Author, speaker and public health advocate.

This practical plan is inspired by the results of Dr. Anne Seifert's National Institutes of Health study to discover how healthy people stay healthy. In 1974 she became co-investigator at the Institutes of Health Research, Pacific Medical Center, in San Francisco. It became clear to her after years of investigation that what we had always suspected was true: sensible eating, moderate exercise, eating breakfast, and sleeping 7 to 8 hours a night were associated with good health and well-being.

What was surprising was how few people were able to change their behavior patterns to achieve the goal of good health. Responsible programs for weight-loss and exercise were often too demanding. Dr. Anne reasoned that if she could find a way to make nutritious well-balanced eating easy and exercise enjoyable, perhaps more people would do it. Not only would people feel better, but they'd also lose weight reducing the risk for many chronic diseases often attributed to old age, including heart disease, diabetes, and cancer.

She concluded that a major culprit eroding good health is excess weight. The MagicHand eating plan was developed to be permissive, allowing people to still eat their favorite foods for a lifetime of healthy eating. Other dally practices were also included— exercise and meditation— completing this overall good health package.

Her first public workshop introducing the hand as a measurer to gauge portions took place on February 6, 1984 for the City of Escondido. Her first book describing the hand measure was published in 1982. Now Dr. Anne can be found online presenting talks to various groups and organizations. She can be reached at www.dranne.org

Acknowledgments

Thank you to all the Practice Circle Members

For showing me that this program really works and inspiring me to keep preaching since my very first class for the City of Escondido in 1984!

Many friends were at my side:
A special thanks to Anne Yedval West for editing my prose. She made this book stronger and leaner. Truly a wonderful gift from a friend.
My husband Fred provided insights, questioned, and listened to my musings.
Actress Renee Aubry promoted our presentations at many Screen Actor's Guild Hollywood events. Greatly appreciated.
My sister Louise attended Practice Circle meetings on my behalf.
Marilyn Goettsch and Sandra Kaminsky led numerous Practice Circles
and Caara VanMerlin was always there for continued support.

Thank you.

Table of Contents

The word *Practice*:
To do or perform frequently— to create a habit.
It is also the act of continually doing something in order to get better at it.

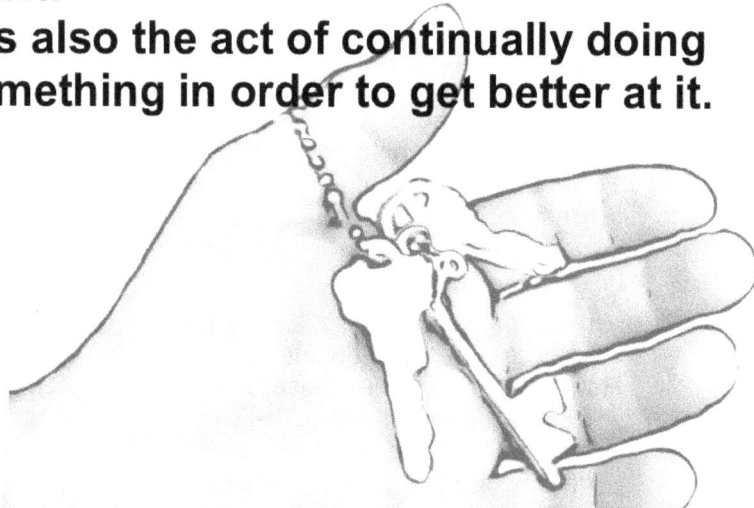

- An example of practice is when you play the piano for 1/2 hour every day to become a better piano player.

Introduction
Three keys to good health

As an epidemiologist, I have studied disease and risk factors predisposing one to disease. It is clear from my years of research that lifestyle counts. Health practices contribute to, mitigate, or avert many chronic diseases. That is the master key: behavior. Clearly, being overweight exacerbates most chronic diseases. This book focuses on keeping your weight under control, staying active, and also finding quiet time. In short, this is a training course on how to live well.

How often have you heard that diets don't work? Well, for the most part, they do! The problem with most restrictive diet regimens is that they are too difficult to incorporate into one's life. Some are able to live with "no-fat" diets, others can abstain from all sugar— they are rare, committed, disciplined people and I applaud them. Most of us still want a brownie.

This book offers a relatively easy and flexible program. Changing habits and finding your own way is the challenge. Imagine that you are about to learn how to play the violin. Someone hands you this instrument, already formed from wood with a bridge and strings and a bow. The objective is to be able to play pleasing music. But first you must learn how. Just as you must learn good health practices.

Your instrument is your body and it came with already set genes and predispositions. Learning the sheet music, and getting that violin to perform as it should requires PRACTICE.

Learning to make music requires coordination between the instrument and player. Practice, Practice, Practice. It does not stop. What musician, even when a virtuoso, stops practicing? And that's what you must do. Never stop practicing to keep good health habits in place. Here is the sheet music, the blueprint, for good health. Keep in mind that perhaps not every day will you be perfect, you may miss a note. It only means you must *keep practicing*.

This book is divided in three parts:

APPORTION   describes how to keep healthy weight control.

MOVE   tells how to find joyful exercising.

SILENCE   instructs how to use meditation to visualize results.

Each part contains three Point chapters for lifelong well-being— staying in tune. Ending each chapter is a Practice page to help you personalize your journey to good health.

How to Use this Book

Chapter Points instruct the reader to take action. You may or may not already have many good habits in place. For example, some people already reserve time for meditation whereas others say they have no time. Read each Point chapter and decide if the subject applies to you. Regardless, answer the questions on the Practice page. You will get the most from this book if you read every Point and complete each Practice.

Practice: At the end of each chapter a Practice page follows to address some issues relevant to the Point. You can complete this section by yourself or discuss your answers with friends in a Practice Circle.

Practice Circle: I recommend at least three people to start a Practice Circle. (See *Appendix C* for details.) If you want to open your Circle to others, list your group on the internet and start a Zoom or other online meeting. Going through the Practice questions with others will help give you the support you need to live the program. After you finish all nine Points, repeat the Points again and again. You will find that each time you repeat the process you will learn something new about yourself. Being with others lends support and keeps you motivated.

APPORTION

Point 1: Measure
Point 2: Hold
Point 3: Adapt

Wave your wand!

Point 1 : Measure

In my work as an epidemiologist I discovered risk factors associated with disease, particularly such chronic diseases as heart disease, diabetes, and cancer. I learned that the one risk factor that exacerbated a present problem and eroded good health is being overweight. I concluded that the major contribution I could make towards public health was to focus on prevention—to create an easy to learn, lifelong approach for maintaining good health and a healthy weight.

The long term solution is committing to a lifetime of good habits. Many have been misled by fad diets or pre-packaged products. After the quick-result diet they return to their prior weight-gain eating.

If you are now overweight forgive yourself. Maybe you don't know, never learned, and were not brought up to eat correctly. We will correct that. I promise this will be an easy and quick-start training course with no frills. You're on your way!

In my first healthy diet book (1982) I brought to national attention the concept of using your hand to visually measure food portions. Many other programs have adopted this idea since then but this program remains the first and only program relying completely on the hand for food measure. It is imprecise making it nutritionally variable but much easier to use than any other program. There's a trade-off I was willing to make between a program being livable yet acknowledging nutritional guidelines, or a program being exacting and strictly following Recommended Daily Allowances (RDA). It also had to be flexible— adaptable to changes in Federal nutritional recommendations and adaptable to medically restricted diets. Olympic level top health is a great goal, but good health is more readily achieved. This is every day livable! However, Practice is key.

You will soon learn how to use what Dr. Anne calls the MagicHand to gauge portion sizes for weight-loss and weight-control in this very first Point chapter. It's a hand trick that works like "magic" to produce results. And your hand is with you wherever you go!

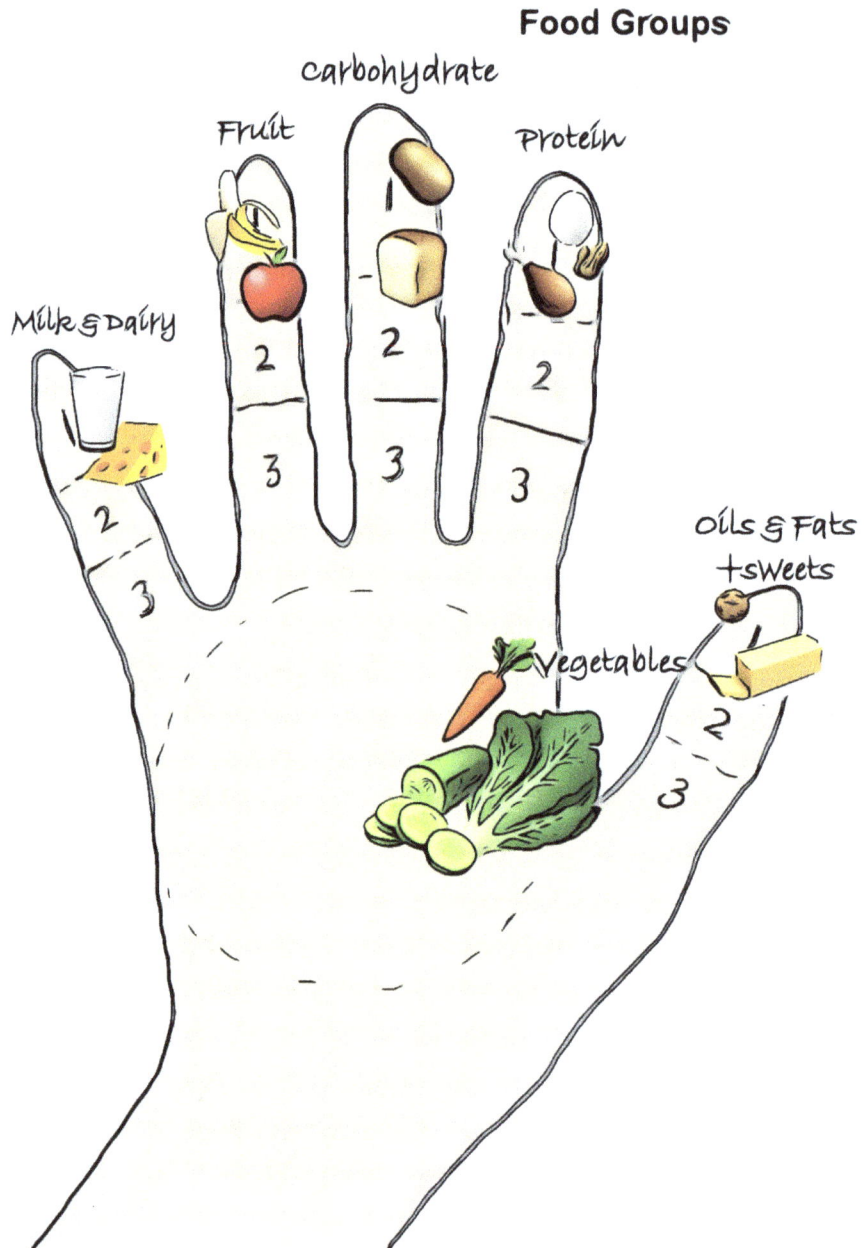

Food Groups

Carbohydrate

Fruit

Protein

Milk & Dairy

2

2

2

3

3

3

Oils & Fats
+ Sweets

2

3

Vegetables

2

3

But first, please take a quick survey. Record for about three days what you eat: for breakfast, lunch and dinner, and make sure to include all snacks. Let's see how your eating changes after you use your MagicHand.

The Quick-Start: Creating your MagicHand

It is time for you to create your own *magic,* that is your MagicHand. Do you agree that to keep weight under control you need to limit portion sizes? Do you agree that to stay healthy it's a good idea to eat a variety of foods? Say yes to both.

You will now learn to use your hand to govern portion-sizes and you will use your fingers to categorize food groups. You may recall from classes in nutrition that food groups are important for a balanced diet. Different foods contribute essential vitamins, minerals and nourishment. Let's start!

Get these materials in front of you: an 81/2" X 11" thick sheet of paper, a good drawing pencil or pen, and five approximately penny-sized round magnets (available at some hardware or craft stores).

Make the drawing following the steps below and write your name at the top. (Or copy and use the illustration in the pages ahead as a model.)

<u>(your name)</u> 's MagicHand.

Now make sure the sheet of paper lies flat. Place your left hand, palm down on the sheet of paper. Place your hand so that there is enough room between the fingers to draw around them. Take your pen and trace your left hand palm down. (Your pinky should be on the left and thumb on the right.)

Draw a light circle inside the palm of your hand so that you will see your palm-size. Divide and number each finger into 3 sections and include the thumb. Start from the top of the finger and number 1, 2, and 3.

Above each finger write the name of the food group that belongs there. Darken the "V" area between your index finger and thumb so that you will remember that this is an open area (for "unlimited Vegetables").
Attach your MagicHand to a metal surface (refrigerator, file cabinet, etc.) and place all the magnets inside your palm circle.

There you have it! Six food groups in your daily menu and a way to control portion size for five of them. But, there's more.

How do I use my MagicHand? Pay attention! Reread this section as many times as needed to learn. The fingers above the palm represent those food groups measured in palm-portions: **the size of that circle inside your palm, and not thicker than the widest part of your thumb.** Or a cupped portion: the amount that would fit inside your cupped hand.

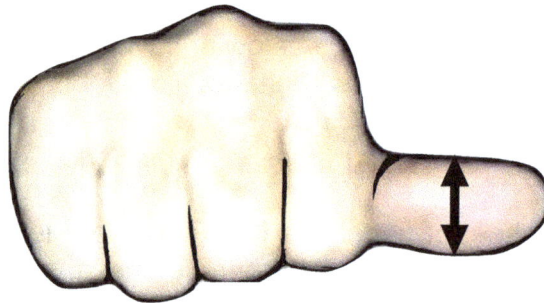

Palm-Portions for each food group: 3 Milk & Dairy, 3 Fruits, 3 Carbohydrates, 3 Proteins. Thumb portions are smaller: 3 Oils & Fats (and sweets). This portion size is **no thicker than the widest part of your thumb.**

(Your name)_____'s *MagicHand*

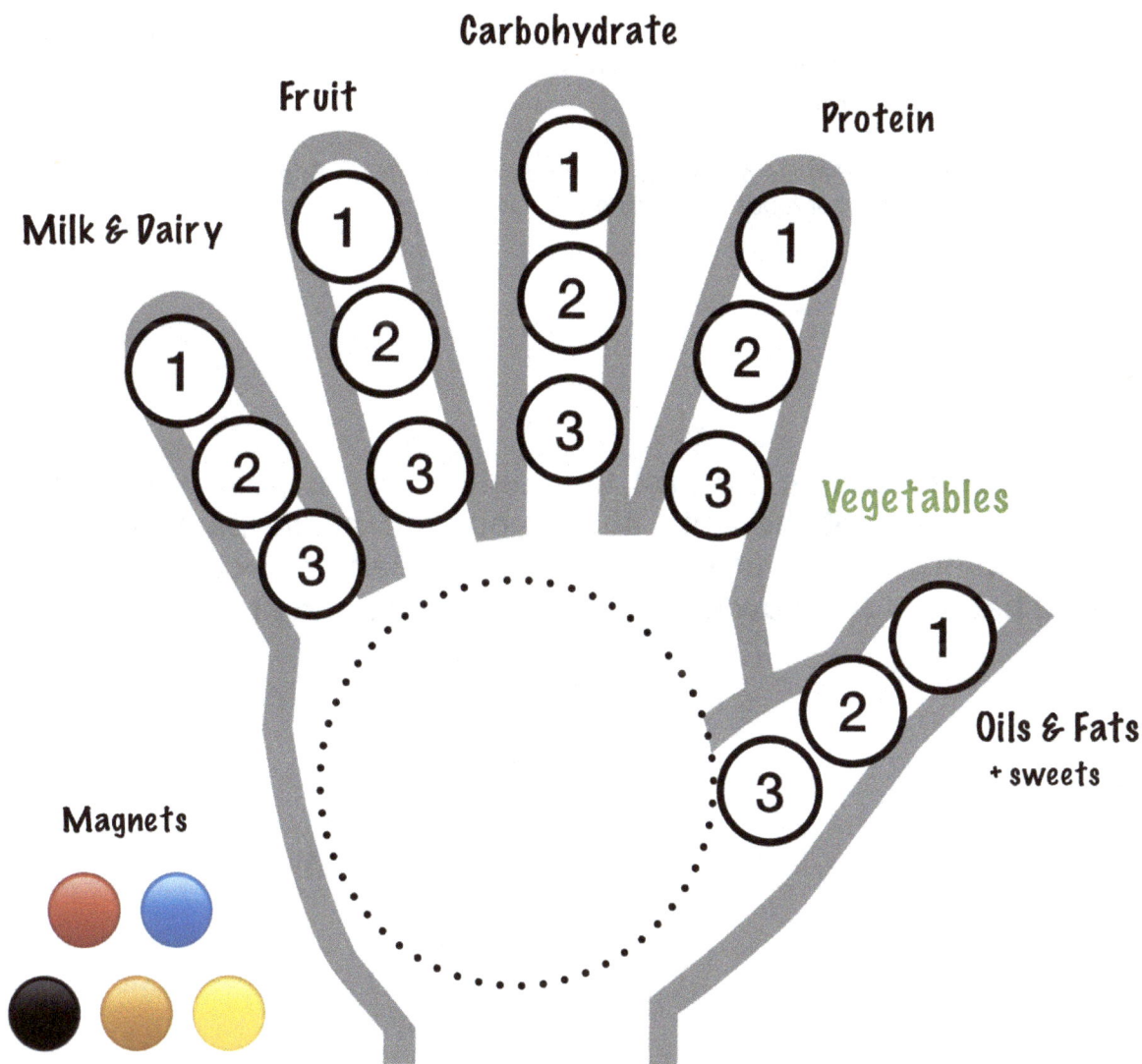

Carbohydrate

Fruit

Protein

Milk & Dairy

1

1

1

1

1

2

2

2

2

3

3

3

3

Vegetables

1

2

3

Oils & Fats
+ sweets

Magnets

Your daily menu consists of 15 MagicHand portions. Vegetables are unlimited. Remember there are only five food groups that need to be counted. This is a **visual** measure for most foods. Of course, an apple can be placed directly in your hand...but not cooked rice!

When you eat, count each portion; place the magnet-counter on your hand drawing on the correct finger food group. When you reach the third portion on the finger, that's it for that food group, for that day.

To understand these measures in standard equivalents See Appendix A.
To see what foods are in different food groups see Appendix E.

Take away message: Control food intake using palm and thumb portioning. Accept the truth about yourself: In the past you were unable to maintain your ideal weight. You can correct and change eating habits— you now know how to eat for the rest of your life!

PRACTICE

Getting to know your Finger foods:
What foods do I really like to eat? List those foods and identify the food group in which they belong: (Milk&Dairy, Fruit, Carbohydrate, Protein, Oils&Fats, or Vegetables) *If needed see* Appendix E for Food Group identity.

Example: _____ice cream__   Food group: Milk & Dairy

_____   _____

_____   _____

_____   _____

_____   _____

_____   _____

_____   _____

_____   _____

_____   _____

How would you measure the portion size for each one listed?

_____

Variety is the spice of life!

Point 2: Hold

The definition of a chit
We call each palm-portion or thumb portion a "chit". You can count "chits" as vouchers. For an entire day you get 12 palm-size chits and 3 thumb size chits. A total of 15 chits each day.

These chits act as "advances" towards your eating budget. Again, you have 15 chits for the day: use them wisely. Use 3 chits and you have 12 left. AFTER you have reached your goal weight your MagicHand chits allotment for the day can become more flexible by making food group portion trades. For example, you could trade a Milk&Dairy chit to get an extra Protein chit. The objective here is to maintain your success, to *hold* your ideal weight.

And yes, you can eat cake
Are you destined for a life of food group monitoring and palm-portion counting? The answer is yes and no. The purpose of using your MagicHand is to teach you how to function like a person who eats well, but also does not gain weight. Since your hand is always with you and you now have been taught to eat "with your eyes" to visualize portion size, you can go anywhere and use your *hand measure*.

This system is extremely adaptable to all situations, but you must learn how to use it so that you can live this way and not feel deprived. After you have reached your ideal weight, the challenge facing you is to maintain that weight, that dress or suit size, that wonderful feeling of being light for the rest of your life. The difference between losing weight and maintaining weight is that when you are losing weight you must choose healthy fiber-rich foods in those palm-portions. Your fruit must be an apple, not a fruitcake!

After you have reached your ideal weight
You can allow yourself to opt for more calorie-dense choices— but still in palm or thumb sized portions. You can also engage in what I call "controlled cheating". Borrow a chit from one food group and use it in another. But remember that the more you do that, the more your healthy diet becomes unbalanced.

How to stretch your palm-portions
How can you "stretch" ice cream? Add a ½ chit of Fruit to your ½ chit for Milk. How can you "stretch" spaghetti? This is my favorite way to do it. One palm of uncooked pasta is what I use (and some judgment is involved). After cooking, it looks like more, but it still counts as 1 palm-chit. Layer a vegetable like spinach or spaghetti squash on your plate as much as you want since Vegetables are "unlimited". Spread the pasta on top. Add tomato sauce. (If it has oil use 1 Oil & Fat chit for that.). Add 1 cupped palm of Parmesan cheese (count 1 Milk chit for that). There you have it! A delicious spaghetti dinner for 3 chits. See *Appendix B* for some sample recipes.

Learn how to juggle your chits!
What happens when your Mother comes to visit bringing your favorite homemade cookies? You'll need to see how many chits you have remaining for that day. If you've used all your chits from the Carbohydrate finger, then it's time to make a trade. Two cookies that fit in your palm may not be enough. Take a chit from another food group. That's okay as long as you stay within the allotted 15 chits budget for the day. The idea is not to feel deprived— to feel that you can eat something that you really want to eat. And if you find you want to use all your chits to consume all the cookies, do so! The next day you might feel sick, but you did stay with the program.

How could this program possibly work? It seems imprecise!
The answer: It works using the "law of averages".
The idea here is to provide you with a lifelong healthy eating plan that allows you to maintain a good weight and balanced nutrition. It is not perfect. Perfectly balanced eating, unless you are in a hospital, is nearly impossible to achieve. Remember the closer you stay to strictly using 3 chits in each food group daily, the better the balance. The less refined sugar, the better the nutrition.

Some days you will eat high nutrient-dense foods; some days you may eat low nutrient-dense foods. Obviously nutrient-dense foods are preferred. But, as long as you keep to the chit allowance and follow the palm and thumb rules, you will keep your weight under control. Keep in mind that ideally the chit portions are 100 calories or less. The important tenet is to keep the palm or thumb portion size and understand that nutrition and calories will vary. But, as in nature, it is the law of averages that keeps our planet and the animal kingdom alive.

.

Please know that your body stores most vitamins & minerals-- and if needed supplies them on demand. As a safety net that your body stores are adequate, I consider a daily multivitamin & mineral supplement that follows RDA (Recommended Daily Allowance) guidelines beneficial. However, high-doses of vitamins or minerals can create imbalances, become toxic, and I advise against that-- unless there is a clear deficiency not responding to RDA, and that diet can't correct.

Time off

Most people who are *not* conscious about what and how much they eat, tend to gain weight. It is for this reason that every day you will be counting chits. Move your magnets on the hand drawing to count chits (portions) as you eat and your day progresses.

However, there are special occasions where you may just say: "The heck with it!" Allow yourself that option. Choose some days for yourself that are totally free of chit-counting. For example: your birthday and Thanksgiving.

Select nine days each year. Select the days beforehand as best you can. That doesn't mean you go crazy with eating on those days. It just means that this program allows for special occasions making it "livable", and that you can follow all the precepts without ruining your good health.

Take away message: After you've had some success, make sure to "hold" that weight loss. It is just as important to maintain your new weight as it was to lose. Do not take too many liberties.

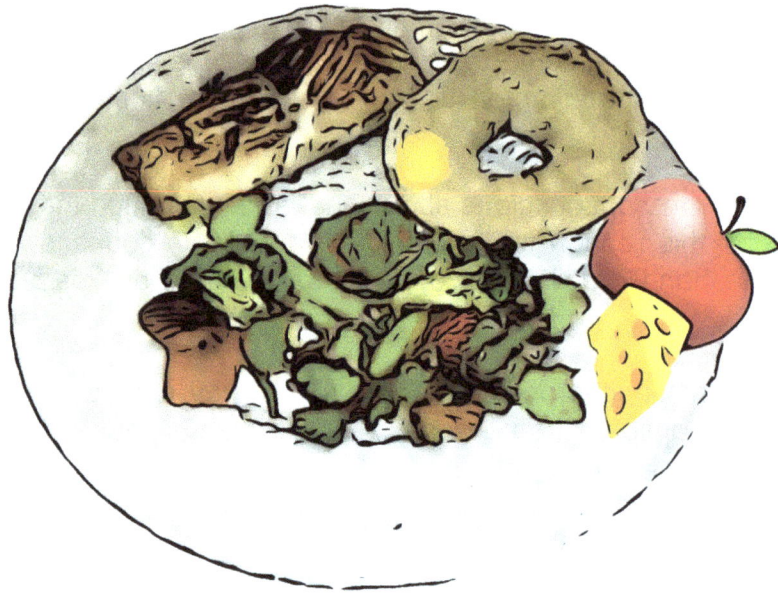

Find the 6 food groups!

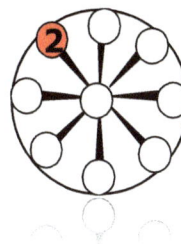

PRACTICE

Think about your favorite foods. How could you "stretch" those portions?
Identify the foods you could "stretch" by adding Vegetables:

_____. _____. _____.

_____. _____. _____.

What food group do I want to eat the most? _____

Is there one food group I don't like at all? _____

Could I meet the nutritional benefit of that food group in some other way?

_____

You can modify your MagicHand by trading the chits from one food group to another. But the more you deviate, the less balanced the diet, and perhaps the more likely for weight gain. How many food group "trades" do you think you could make without gaining weight?

_____

_____

Minefields ahead!

Point 3: Adapt

The good news is that wherever you go you will have your hand, the measurer, with you. No counting calories, adding up grams, or weighing foods! BUT the bad news is that you will have to remember how many palm-portions you are taking with you to the party. In Point 3 we will answer the question: how can I *handle* eating away from home?
You will learn how to plan ahead for special events and holidays and how to eat at restaurants. You will learn how to count your chits!

Plan ahead
Plan for parties and special events by modifying your intake (saving chits) at other meals during the day. You cannot save chits from a previous day or plan not to eat as much the next day. Every day must stand on its own two feet and be governed by your hand! The rule is: 12 finger-palm food portions and 3 thumb-joints a day, and unlimited vegetables.

Everyone has a way of modifying intake. Some people skip breakfast, which I don't recommend if it makes you too hungry. For after-dinner parties I usually forego one milk and my starch and fat at dinner time anticipating the foods that are likely to tempt me at a party. For dinner I'll have my protein portion and an almost full plate of vegetables which I find very satisfying and filling. (I may drink some milk just before I leave for the party if it will take the edge off of any hunger.). Grapefruit juice is good as a hunger-quencher too.

At the party, I will eat the Carbohydrate that (visually) fits in the palm of my hand. This could mean some crackers or puff pastry. You **can** make trades and once you become practiced in the system, your eating habits can be easily governed.

Inevitably you will encounter people who encourage you to eat more even when they know that you are in the process of losing weight. Prepare yourself for dealing with these saboteurs. Recognize it for what it is and resolve to win. If this person is your husband, wife or someone else close to you, there may be other issues that need to be addressed as well. You need to put the control and power on your side when it comes to your own eating. Let them "win" somewhere else if it's that important, but not on **your** plate!

Fast-food restaurants, dinner dates, traveling, partying, and coffee klatches need not throw you off your diet anymore. Use your head as well as your hand. Excesses of food, family traditions, and accompanying feelings at social events outside your home can be safely negotiated. It takes *practice*.

Fast Foods
Dissecting your hamburger into portions can be a challenge. Depending on the size of your burger, it could be 2 Carbohydrate chits for the bun and 1 Protein chit for the meat. Add a slice of cheese and that's a ½ Milk chit.

Count your chits and enjoy. Do not concern yourself about how the food was prepared, whether fried or baked or grilled. A palm portion of French fries is still 1 Carbohydrate chit. We are not counting calories. Calories will vary from day to day— BUT on average, you will be consuming 1200-1500 calories per day on this program.

Traveling
In the car: Have on hand some "snack packs" so you don't get hungry and need to pull over for fast-food. Having trail mix, V-8 juice, maybe a banana, might keep you satisfied. Make a pack for your car and keep it on hand.
On trains and planes: Often portions tend to be small so it many not be as difficult to keep on track. Use your common sense. Drink plenty of water to stay hydrated.

Restaurants
This is the biggest challenge. Portion sizes tend to be very large. Immediately plan for the doggie bag. Cut the meat portion in half (if over-sized). Eat all the vegetables and salad. Save some chits in advance for this event. Have the dessert you want, or split the dessert, or have none at all. Sometimes coffee at the end of a meal is just as good.

Part of the restaurant dinner could be tomorrow's lunch!

Holidays

Some holidays might be days to select as part of the program's recommended 9-day/year chit-free days. November and December are the tough months and it is not unusual for the average person to gain from 4-7 pounds over just those two months. But you will be on guard, counting chits. What I do is "save chits" during the day if I know I will be attending a holiday party or event. I bring my hand with me, and count as I am offered hors d'oeuvres. I count the beverages (⅓ cup of alcohol beverage = 1 chit). Juggle your chits, eat what you like, and stay within that budget.

Learn the phrases of the "skinny people" who know how to say 'no'. Use the phrases: "I'd like some but I'm just too full". "Oh, just a little piece, I'm stuffed". "Thank you, I'll have some later".

As a houseguest

Where you really lack control is in someone's home! Depending on how well you know your host, you could make some special requests, join them on a food shopping trip, or bring a basket of goodies (fruits & nuts) with you as a house gift. Again, count your chits and do not worry about balancing all the food groups. Keep to your 15 portion-chits for the day. If all they serve are donuts for breakfast and sandwiches for lunch and pasta for dinner you will be making food group chit trades. When you return home, a balanced diet with 3 chits per food group can be resumed.

Take away message: You can adapt your MagicHand to special circumstances and occasions in order to maintain your ideal weight. Learn by trial and error.

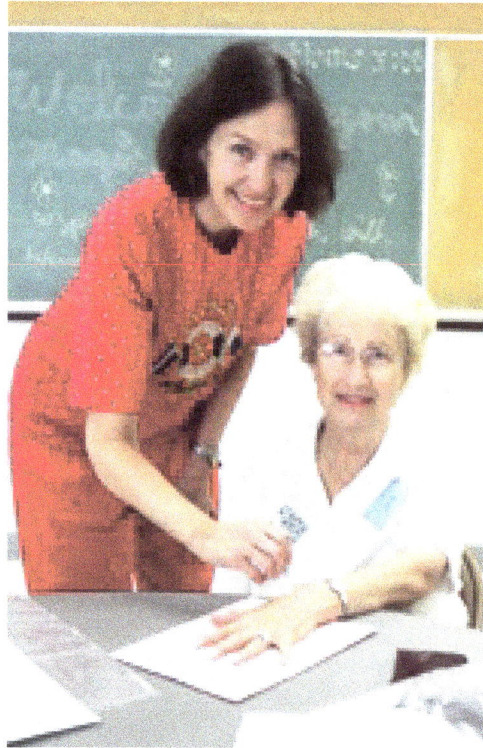

Drawing the MagicHand

PRACTICE

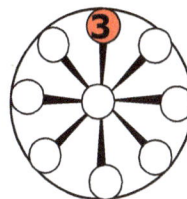

Go through your calendar starting in January. What days for sure will you not be counting chits? (You have 9 no-chit days each year).

_____. _____. _____

_____. _____. _____

_____. _____. _____

How will you say "no" to people who try to push food on your plate?
Give a quote:

_____

_____

How many chits will you bring with you if you eat at a restaurant?

_____.

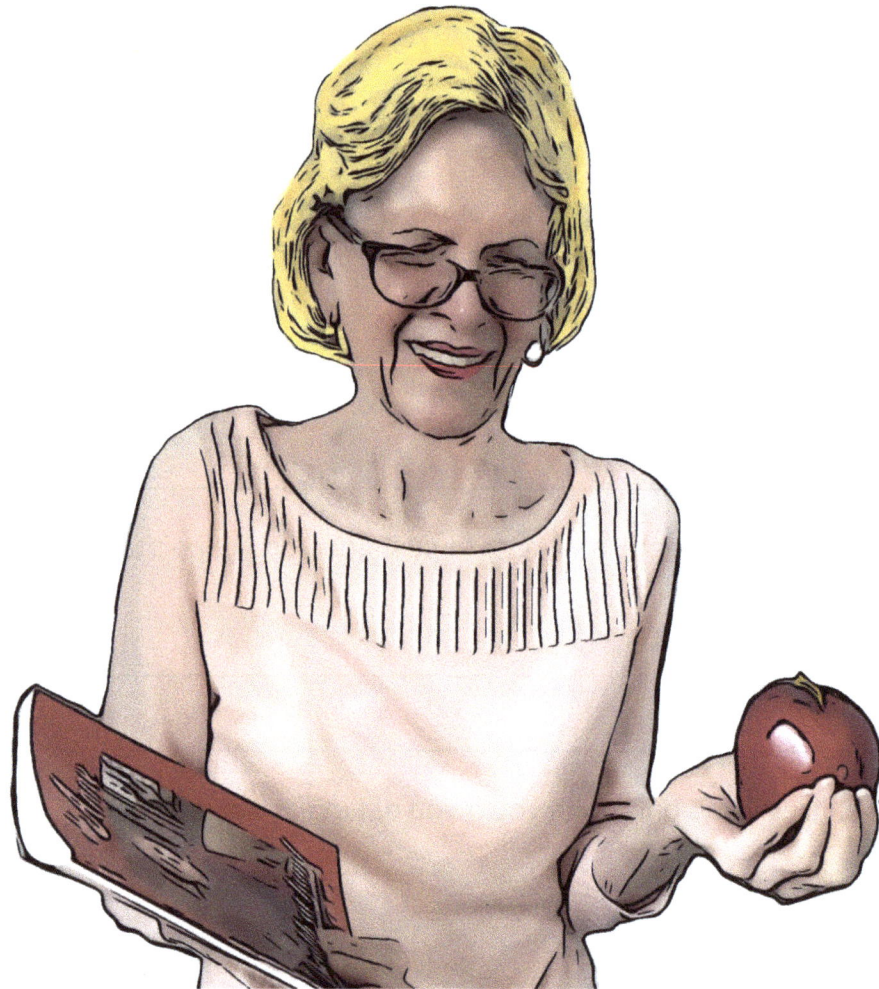

Practice!

MOVE

Point 4: Goals
Point 5: Play
Point 6: Control

You're on your way!

Point 4: Goals

Do you have the answer to this question: What is my ideal weight?
To answer that question it might be helpful to remember the "you" that once was at a very desirable weight. If there never was that time, think of what weight would make you happy now. What clothing size would you like to maintain for the rest of your life?

Look for either a photo of yourself at your desired weight or a picture in a magazine of your goal body shape and size. Post that photo where you can see it every day. A wardrobe closet door perhaps.

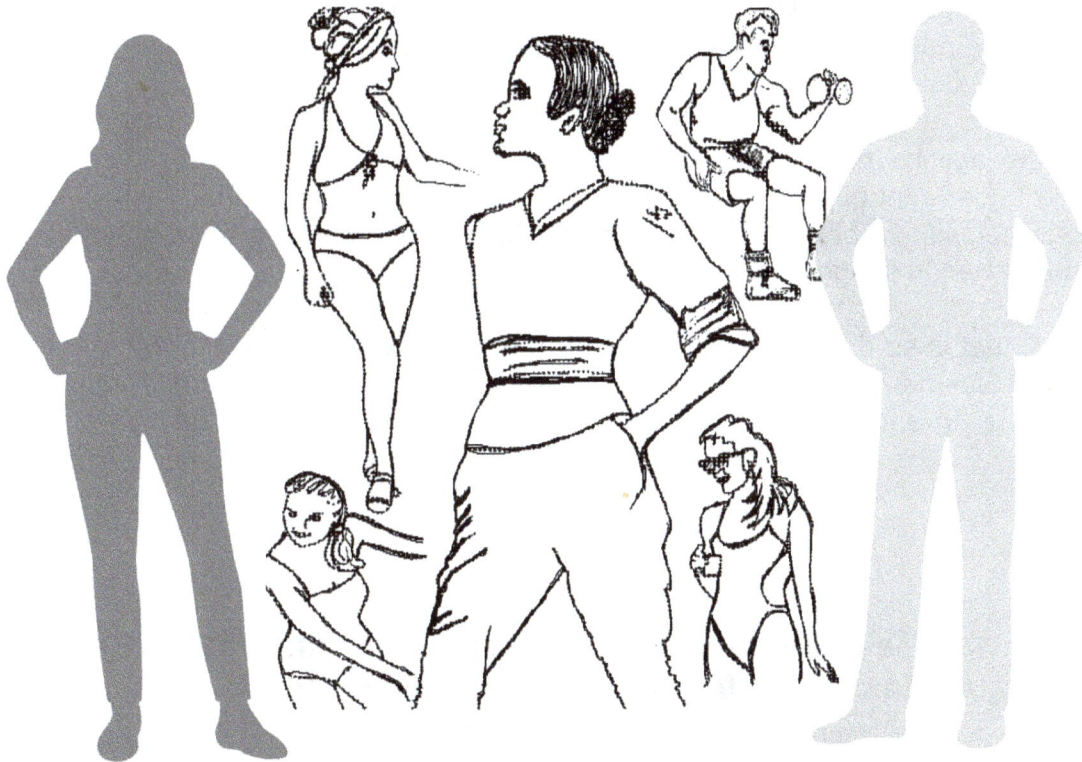

Now take your ideal weight number and add two pounds; then take your ideal weight number and subtract two pounds. This is your "ideal weight range". The goal is to stay in the middle. If you reach the top of that range it's time to get strictly back to your MagicHand eating. No trades. Make the commitment to stay in that weight range once you reach your ideal weight. Promise.

Make it a ritual to record your weight at least once a month. If you need support find a "buddy" to report your weight loss progress. This will keep you accountable. Remember that it may take a while for those extra pounds to disappear. And there are daily fluctuations up and down. Weigh yourself as often as you wish but only record your weight once a month. This way you can see your progress. Looking back at what you have accomplished is motivating and inspiring. It is also helpful to notice the times when you either gained or lost weight. In either case try to analyze what happened in your life at that time. Soon you will have your personal history of weight loss and gain patterns. Well-balanced eating and natural weight-loss is the goal.

Your old actions need to be changed. Those who have problems keeping their weight under control just cannot be given free rein. It is unlikely that you will ever be able to eat without being conscious of your intake. And keeping track of your weight alerts you when to tighten the reins!

The pill that is so difficult to swallow is that the permanent correction of your weight requires lifetime commitment. You maybe don't know or never learned or were not brought up to eat correctly. New habits must replace the old. And again, it takes *practice.*

Take away Message: Record your weight monthly, make notes— you'll soon learn how to maintain your ideal weight!

PRACTICE

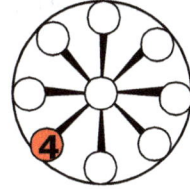

Think about the 'body you want'. Visualize it, and find a picture to place where you can see it daily.

Record your "ideal weight range". (-2lbs.=_____ Ideal=_____ +2lbs.=_____)

Can   you see yourself at your "ideal weight"? _____

Any exercise is better than no exercise!

Point 5: Play

For a healthy body muscles need to move and heart and lungs need to be worked more than usual. It is difficult to lose weight just through exercise. But without it you will probably not be able to maintain good health or your ideal weight.

Since some people react negatively to the word exercise, let's call it physical play. Certainly as a child you had fun "playing".   Most likely that playing involved a physical sport. Let's go back to that time.

Did you play hopscotch?   When it snowed did you go sledding? Or did you stay inside and dance to music? When summer arrived, did you go to the beach? What was your "fun"?

All you really need to do is find one sport or activity that you find appealing. I like to swim, I like to ride my bicycle, and for most of the year, I like to walk. For many, walking is the easiest exercise. When you do walk, stand straight and if unsteady on your feet, I recommend using walking sticks aka trekking poles. You can become mediocre in a large number of sports and still enjoy them! In short, the best exercise for you is the one you'll do consistently and enjoy.

Here's the rule for whatever play activity you select: Make sure to **'exercise' every other day for 30 minutes**. You can do more if you wish, but not less to maintain fitness.

Start slowly. In addition, do this simple exercise to strengthen your back and abdominal muscles to avoid injury.

The pelvic tilt:
Lie on your back, bend your knees with feet planted on the ground. Relax. Breathe in, expanding your belly. Tighten your buttocks, pull in your belly muscles to press your lower spine flat to the floor as you exhale to a slow count of five.

Release all the muscles. Now do it again!

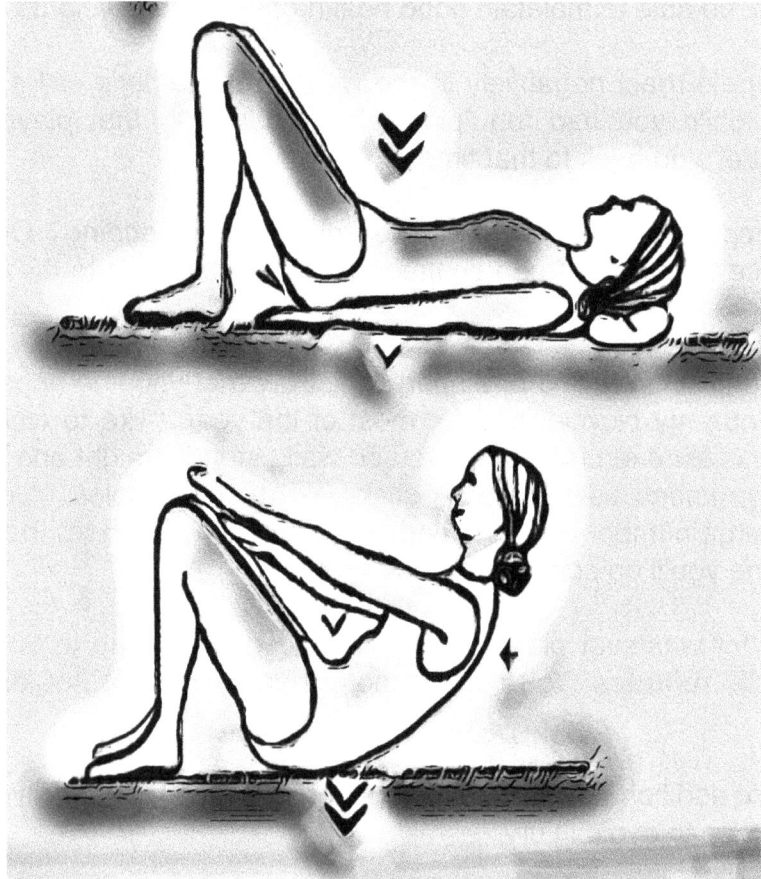

Stand and check your body alignment. Are you standing straight, even? Look in the mirror, side view. Pull in those abdominals. Look at your feet when you walk. Toes straight. Make sure your heels hit the ground first!

Develop a contingency plan for alternate physical play activities if the weather or circumstances change, not permitting your regular activity.

Be sure to have the appropriate equipment for your physical play activity. Read books for pointers on your sport or take lessons from an expert who will not push you too quickly.

Start your physical play program slowly, especially if you are overweight. If you are more than 10 pounds overweight, proceed cautiously. Plan to play once a week at first, and then graduate to twice a week and so on until you reach the physical play guidelines of at least every other day. Take it one step at a time.

Take away message: Find an exercise that you enjoy and make it your physical play! Commit to at least 30 minutes every other day.

Physical Play Ideas
Check the ones you "like" without thinking of exercise benefits. Add others if you wish. Select at least one activity for each season! And one for indoors!

aerobic dancing	fitness trail	raquetball	table tennis
Aikido/Tai chi	flexibility exercises	roller skating	tap dancing
archery	football/touch	rope skipping	tennis
badminton	frisbee	rowing	trampoline/mini
ballet	gardening	rugby	treadmill
baseball/softball	golf	running/jogging	volleyball
basketball	gymnastics	sailing/yachting	walking
bicycling	handball	scuba/skin diving	water skiing
bocce ball	hiking/backpacking	shuffleboard	weight lifting
boogieboard	hockey/ field/ice	skateboarding	
bowling	horseback riding	skiing/ downhill	
boxing/wrestling	ice/figure skating	snowboarding	
calisthenics	judo/karate	snowshoeing	
canoeing	kayaking	soccer	
cricket	lacrosse	spinning	
cross country skiing	mtn. climbing	square dancing	
dancing/ ballroom	paddle ball	squash	
diving	pickleball	surfing/ board/ wind	
fencing	polo	swimming	

PRACTICE

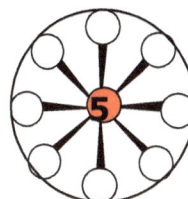

Write down your favorite sports or outdoor activities: (think about at least one for each season).

_____._____._____._____
Summer. *Fall.* *Winter.* *Spring*

What do you need to get started now? (Equipment, facilities, etc.) Any obstacle to overcome?

_____

_____

What would be an alternative 'physical play' if it rains, or your practice partner doesn't show up, or you are traveling or something else happens?

_____

_____

When and where will you practice your 'pelvic tilt'?

_____

It's worth your time!

Point 6: Control

A good healthy life requires changes to your allotment of time. Maybe your regular shopping now takes longer because you're picking up heads of lettuce instead of fast food. Maybe finding time to exercise means forgoing some TV. So, how can you find the time to stay healthy?

Time blocks

To organize your day and to be sure that you include time for healthful activities think in blocks of time. Do you know where your time actually goes? One way to find out is to record on a sheet of paper —divided into hour sections— exactly what you are doing each hour. Sometimes it's surprising to discover how much time is spent on phone calls or texting, TV, or running errands.

If you find almost all your time goes to your job you may have to re-evaluate your priorities. Don't sacrifice your health on the altar of work. Easier said than done I know.

Some of these suggestions may help to get extra time in your day:
• Set time limits on your activities.
• Consolidate similar activities.
• Identify your peak work performance hours. Do your important tasks then.

What is the actual amount of time needed?

For exercise: At least 30 minutes every other day, is 90-120 minutes/week.
For Meal Planning: A guesstimate is 60 minutes/week.
For Meditation: Each day, minimum of 10 minutes, is 70 minutes/week.

Total time to add healthy living= 220 to 250 minutes or about 4 hours/week.

Somewhere in your busy schedule can you find about 4 hours each week to devote to your good health? What competes for those hours? For most it is family, work, hobbies, television, internet, clubs, distractions, etc. Our lives are busy, complicated, and not without upsets here and there. Look at your day, see what robs your time, and give some time back to yourself for your own well-being.

Take away message: the benefit of good health is worth finding the time to establish good habits. Make it a priority in your life.

PRACTICE

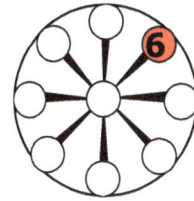

When can I find the time to 'stay healthy'? Evaluate your day. In light pencil sketch in "**pie slices**" showing how you spend your time now. In colored or dark pen— sketch where you can find the time to meditate and exercise and prepare meals.

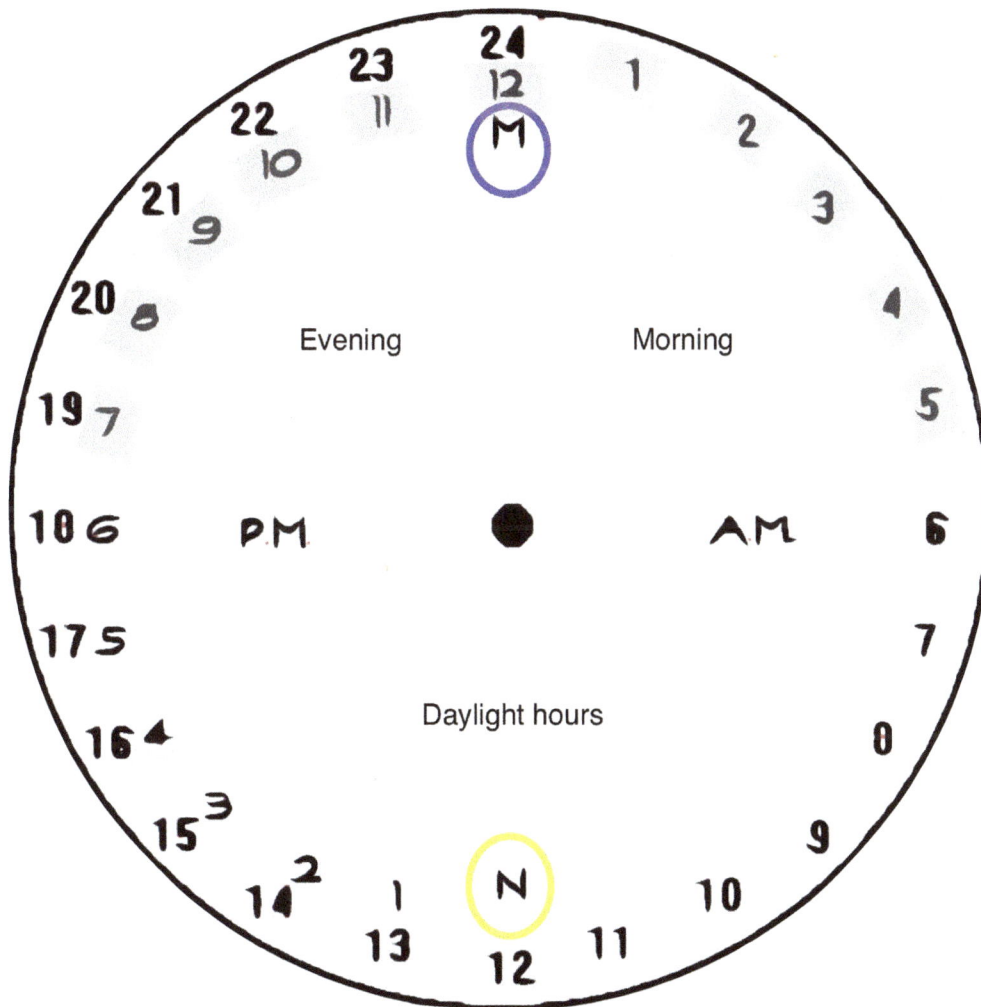

*"It is worthy to perform the present duty well and without failure;
do not seek to avoid or postpone it till tomorrow.
By acting now one can have a good day."*— *Bukkyo Dendo Kyokai*
from "The Teaching of Buddha"

SILENCE

Point 7: Inner
Point 8: Nurture
Point 9: Daily

Feel the feeling.

Point 7: Inner

How do your mind and body interact? Your mind is the director of your body and feelings can contribute to overeating.

The "magic key"
For many the missing key to achieving healthy eating is not a lack of knowledge. Rather, it is the inability to acknowledge feelings which create the 'need' to stuff those feelings! Recognizing when food is a substitute for comfort, love, and friendship is key to healthy eating.

The way you behave, the way you think, and the way you feel directly influences your physical being.

Is your eating style keeping you from successful healthy living and weight control? The three types of eating most likely to be problematic are:

(1) *High intake eating* (that means just eating too much)
(2) *Trigger food eating* (that means certain foods lead to binge eating and
(3) *Stuffing feelings eating* (that means eating when upset or even happy).

For these three styles of unhealthy eating, new behaviors must be substituted and that requires self examination.

For **High intake**— Your physical "appestat" needs to be readjusted. When you feel 80% full stop eating.

For **Trigger food**— Identify your binge foods. These foods can be either psychological or physiological triggers.

For **Stuffing feelings**— Identify your feelings and keep a diary to record them. Find other ways to get comfort or relief from stress. Engage in 'self-talk'.

Ask yourself 'What am I feeling?' Can I find comfort by doing something other than eating? Discover the answers. Take a walk. Smell the roses. Take a bath. Talk to a friend. Be determined.

Make the **decision** to go for victory. Don't stuff. Take action.

Take Away Message:

Get in touch with your feelings and see if they influence your eating. Acknowledge those feelings and find another way to release them.

PRACTICE

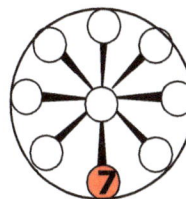

Here's a mental exercise. Make sure to check in with your feelings.

Close your eyes. Visualize yourself at your ideal weight.
Now visualize yourself as you are right now. Keep taking off 5 pounds until you reach your ideal body weight. Ask: Was that weight serving any purpose? If not, release it visually. Let it go. With every 5 pounds released ask yourself: 'How do I feel?'

_____

_____

How would you classify your eating style?
Good, High Intake, Food Trigger Binger, and/ or Stuffing Feelings eater?

_____

For any of the above, is there something you could do differently? If so, what?

_____

_____

Give yourself a break!

Point 8: Nurture

Do you remember when you found time in your day (back at Point 6) for exercise and meal planning? Do you recall that 10 minutes is allotted for daily meditation? This section explores the benefits of meditation and what type of meditation would be best for you.

Almost everyone has some stress in life. Constant stress simply wears you down. Concerns about relationships, finances, work and health probably account for most, if not all, the emotional stress in our everyday living. Many live in fear of failing to mitigate these stressors. Others know how to find peace no matter the issues.

Do you feel loved by yourself or others?   Do you find satisfaction at work and at home? Do you find enough money to pay your bills in your checking account? Examine these three arenas and observe when you feel frustrated, angry or depressed.

To keep an even keel, the magic power of meditation works. We can nourish our psyches through quiet time. It takes a minimum of 10 minutes a day and *practice.* Most people, at first, will find many thoughts rushing through their mind. That is normal. After some practice you will learn to let those thoughts go and allow yourself to drift with 'no thought'. Peace.

One reason that meditation is incorporated into this program is because any change made in your lifestyle even if a healthy change can produce stress.

Meditation is a way to relax, a way to find quiet time.

Meditation calms your mind and allows for an easier transition to new behaviors and good habits. Visualizing and affirming your goals during this time facilitates and supports that process.

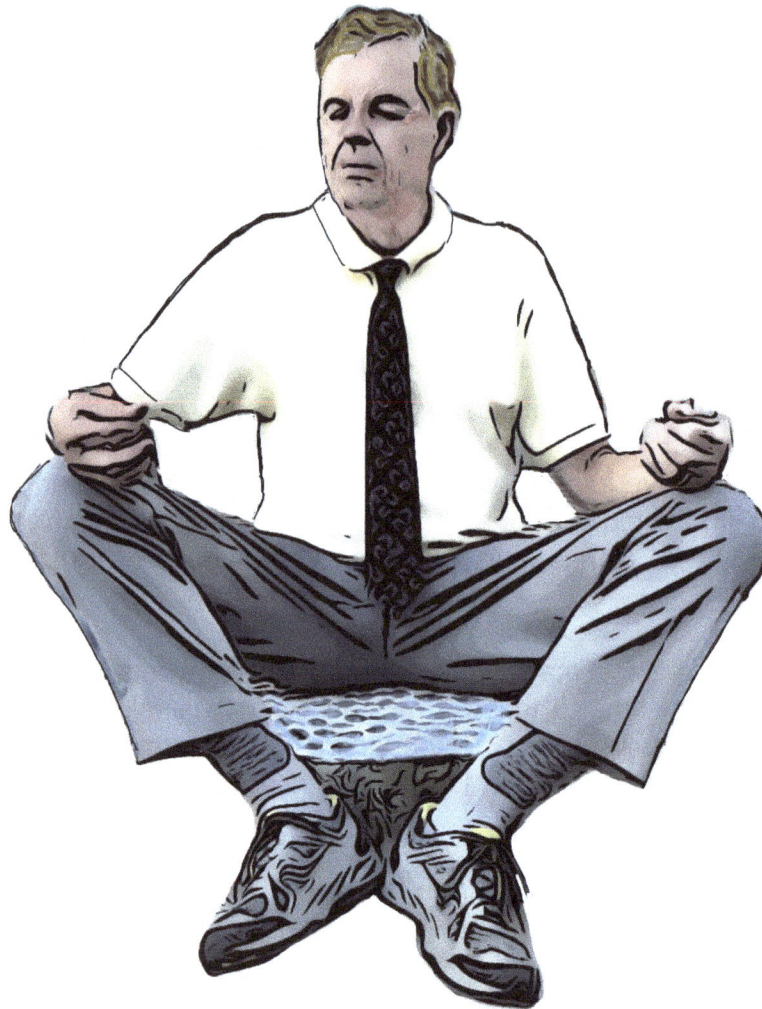

Take away message:
Slow breathing and relaxation contribute to good health. Find the
time to meditate and nurture your soul.

PRACTICE

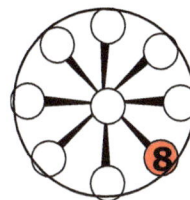

The experience of ten minutes of silence for some people is unsettling because disturbing thoughts that may have been pushed down can surface. Eventually you will be able to overcome recurring thoughts. Remember this silence is healing.

Find a quiet place to sit or lie down. Get comfortable. Set a timer for 10 minutes (or more if you'd like).
Try this meditation exercise:
Close your eyes and breathe slowly, deeply. Concentrate on your breathing. When you feel relaxed visualize yourself and remove five pounds. Keep doing this until you reach your ideal body size or weight.
Say to yourself: "I am now at my ideal weight of _____".

Vary this exercise as you wish to serve your purpose.

Ten minutes of silence often feels very long (which is why the timer is important). However, some people feel that this silence is like taking a "vacation".

What was your experience in these moments of silence?

_____

When are you going to find the time to meditate daily?

_____

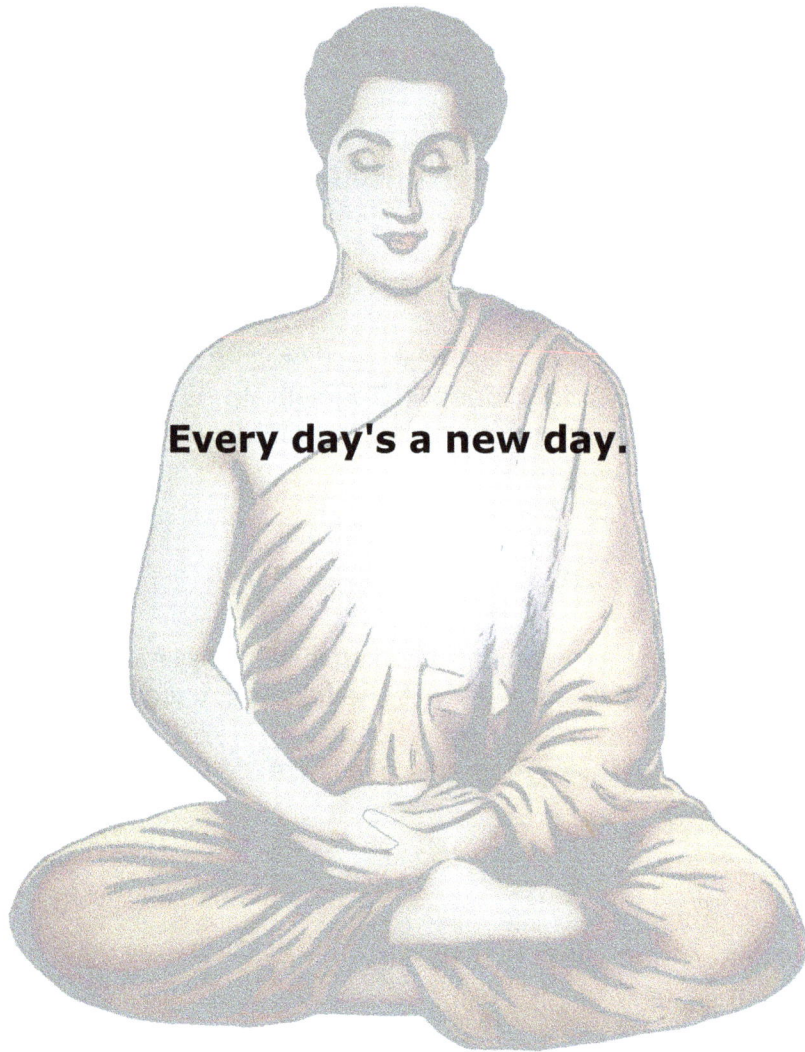

Every day's a new day.

Point 9: Daily

It is your decision to make to change habits and adopt new behaviors for a healthier eating lifestyle. I can make suggestions and provide a blueprint. You have to make the choice and use your power to change. You simply must decide to make it happen and follow through.

Ask yourself these questions over and over again. How can I make this program *my* way of life? How can I make it enjoyable for myself? How can I avoid feeling deprived? When you find the solution to an obstacle, test it.

Hand in hand
My first book on healthy lifestyle was restrictive and many found it too hard (to eliminate foods laden with sugar or saturated fats for example). The second book (MagicHand Eating Plan) was not as restrictive and introduced a "magic" theme since I learned that's what most people want! This, my third health book, is brief, simple, and to the point.

How will you start? If your goal is to lose weight, I suggest strictly following the MagicHand for at least 3 days. See how it feels to eat this way. Can you do that?

This is an investment towards a future full of good health and weight control. If you decide that you can live within the program guidelines then continue to increase the number of days that you strictly follow the program. It takes about 21 days to change a habit. Our minds are constructed in such a way that old habits don't die overnight. Forgive yourself for going backwards if that happens. Every day is a new day. Forge ahead. (See *Appendix D for other ways to count chits*)

Support groups can be helpful. For over 10 years I taught this program in Practice Circle groups. Meetings were held through universities, city recreation departments and in private communities. Just by looking at the faces of attendees I could see the "light bulb" moment when a person made the commitment to follow the program. It's very simple: the program will work once you have decided to do it!

It has been tested and it works. And if you can make a permanent change with another program that fits more with your personal preferences and lifestyle, then do it! Find your own way. This program is moderate, "the middle way".

If you have friends who want to lose weight, form a Practice Circle and meet weekly to discuss each focus Point. You will find that you learn from others and that their support will keep you motivated. See *Appendix C* on how to form your own Practice Circle.

After you have absorbed all nine Points, you should be well practiced on the principles of good health. If you have lost weight following this program, and you have found the program livable, make an even deeper commitment to keep it in place.

If after 21 days of consistently using your MagicHand you have experienced normal healthy eating, and you have lost weight, and you feel good, vow that you will **commit** to keep MagicHand eating in place for **the rest of your life**.

This new pattern of eating will be so rewarding that you will be motivated to maintain your results. Like the violinist, consider yourself in lifelong training. This is a training course for a healthy life. Like any artist or athlete you will always be perfecting your skills and continuing to learn. Practice.

If you lose weight, and then go back to your old way of eating, you can expect to gain back the weight. Don't do it. Be good to yourself. Love yourself well.

This book is a manual "in perpetuity" for good health for the rest of your life. Read it over and over again. Every time you pick up this book it will reinforce good health practices. Commit to read at least two pages every day; leave the book in a place where it's easy to find. Most importantly with these guidelines *Find Your Own Way* to the health and happiness you deserve.

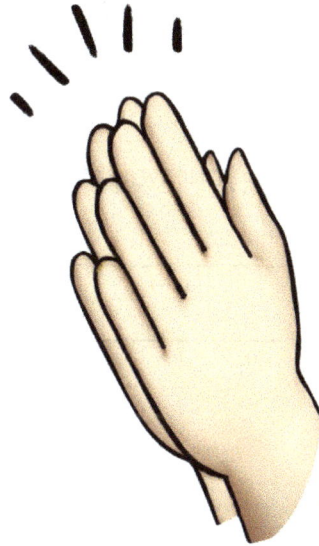

Take away message:
To keep your weight under control follow this program—
** adopt healthy habits for life.**

PRACTICE

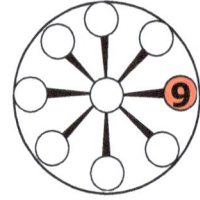

What are your reasons for controlling your weight? Are they good enough for a lifetime?

_____

_____

Are there any obstacles?

_____

How are you going to count your chits? Are you going to use the hand diagram or have you found another way?

_____

Can you commit to living this way for the rest of your life?

_____

Open Sesame!

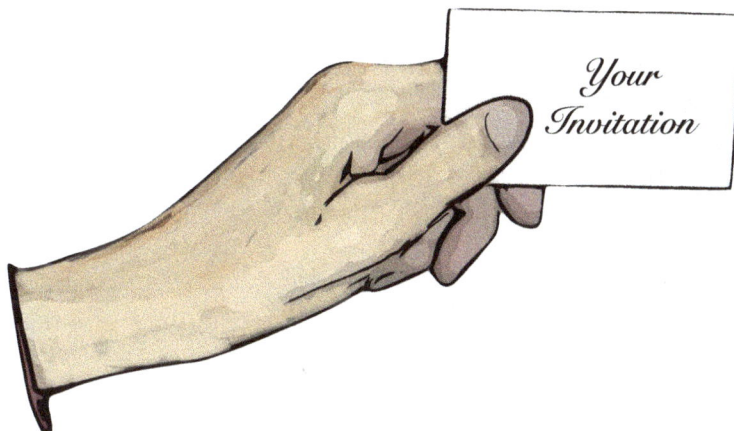

Appendices

A MagicHand Equivalent Measures: Familiar standard measures
B MagicHand Cookery sample
C Practice Circles for Support: Using the MagicSquare
D MagicHand Chits Page: Other ways to tally hand portions
E Seeing Fingers on your MagicHand: Foods under each finger food group

Appendix A
MagicHand EQUIVALENT MEASURES

MagicHand Portion Measure: **STANDARD Measure:**

For Milk & Dairy, Fruit, Carbohydrates and Proteins:

1 Palm-portion that's a spooned or soft food =	2-3 Tablespoons
1 Palm-portion that's liquid=	1/4- 1/2 cup
1 Palm-portion that's rounded & hand held =	1/3 cup
1 Palm-portion that's Thumb thick= 3 in.diameter X 1 in.thick	1-4 oz.

For Oils & Fats:

1 Thumb-joint that's solid=	1 teaspoon
1 Thumb-joint that's soft=	1 teaspoon
1 Thumb-joint of oil or liquid (if watered down)=	1 Tablespoon

For Vegetables:

Unmeasured/ Unlimited

For Sauces, Gravies, Syrups, Stews, Casseroles, Mixed Beverages, Fast Foods, Exotic Desserts, Preserves, Candy, Chocolate and Other unidentified foods:

1 Palm-portion, (sugar/fat laden) liquid, soft or spooned=	2-3 Tablespoons
1 Palm-portion, liquid, rounded, hand-held or cut=	1/4-1/2 cup
1 Thumb-portion (fat/sugar laden) liquid, soft or spooned=	1 teaspoon
1 Thumb-portion (fat/sugar laden) watered down=	1 Tablespoon

When in doubt: Important

Each chit portion ideally should be <u>no more than 100 calories</u>. The default for a cupped palm is 1/3 cup. The less fat and sugar in a palm portion, the fewer the calories. The more fiber in a palm portion, the healthier. MagicHand measures vary due to differences in hand size. STANDARD measures are precise. The hand measure is not perfect, but it works!

Appendix B
MagicHand Cookery sample

Food Group

PITA POCKET MEAL
1 pita bread pocket sandwich	C
1/2 cup alfalfa sprouts	V
1 slice natural low-fat cheese (2 oz.)	M
4 oz. fish or chicken	P
1 t. mayonnaise	O
1 t. mustard	free

Spread mayonnaise and mustard inside pita bread. Stuff with cheese and fish or chicken, and sprouts. Makes 1 serving.
1 serving= 1 Carb chit, 1 Milk chit, 1 Protein chit, 1 Oil chit

MOTHER'S VEGETABLE COMBINATION DISH
4 cups vegetables in season (broccoli, squash, carrots, etc.)	V
1/2 cup natural cheddar cheese, shredded	M
1/2 cup brown rice	C

Cook brown rice and let stand. Steam vegetables for about 15 minutes until just tender. Place the hot vegetables in the center of a large serving place and top with the shredded cheese. While cheese is melting ring the vegetables with rice. Serve immediately. Makes 2 servings.
1 serving= 1 Carbohydrate chit, 1 Milk chit

DEBBIE'S DELIGHT COOKIES
1 1/2 cups whole wheat/oat flour	C
1/2 cup bran	C
1 3/4 cups old fashioned oats	C
1/2 t. baking soda	free
1/2 t. salt	free
1/4 cup cooking oil	free
1/2 cup honey/brown sugar	O
1 egg ,well beaten	P
1 t. vanilla	free
1/2 cup chopped walnuts	P
1 cup mashed over-ripe banana (or applesauce, cooked squash/pumpkin)	F or V
1/2 cup raisins	F

Mix all dry ingredients. Then add all mixed liquids and include banana, walnuts and raisins. Place batter in rounded tablespoons on greased cookie sheet. Bake for 15 minutes in 350 degree oven. Makes about 5 dozen cookies (textured and crunchy). 2 cookies= 1 Carbohydrate chit

Appendix C
Practice Circles for Support

MagicHand Practice Circles operate across the country using a format similar to the one described below. Use this format to form your own self-help Practice Circle!

How to Form a Practice Circle
Here are the steps to follow:
First, you will need to form a **T E A M**:

Three At Least	Participating members to form a group
Experience	Knowledge using the MagicHand
Administrative	Keeping in touch with members
Meeting space	Providing a regular place/time to meet

Secondly, find a place to meet. This could be either in-person (a home, meeting room, or cafe) or online (via Zoom or other internet venue). Establish a time when at least 3 people can meet on a regular basis. Eventually through social media or notices others will join you.

Next, select officers **The Three Linking Hands** and designate responsibilities
Ruling-Hand: Contact phone number and/or email for the Practice Circle.
Right-Hand: Assists the Ruling-Hand, may organize registration events.
Post-Hand: Meeting notices. Donations for group expenses.

If desired: create a space for your Practice Circle on social media.
See **www.dranne.org** website for links and more details.

How to conduct the Meeting:
This book has three sections: <u>Apportion</u>, <u>Move</u>, and <u>Silence</u>. Under each section there are three chapters called Points: a total of nine chapter Points.

Meetings are for support. Keep focused on one Point each meeting using the Practice questions in this book to stimulate discussion. The next meeting then focuses on the following Practice Point. After reaching Point 9, start all over again!

Why is it called a Practice Circle?
New participants can enter at any time. The Points continue, from one meeting to the next meeting, and repeat again. Like a circle, practice and learning are never ending!

Learn to use the MagicSquare for Completing Practice Points:
What is the MagicSquare? (It's on the last page!)
Did you notice that on each Practice page there was a circle in the upper right corner displaying the Point number? That was not just for decoration!

Looking at the MagicSquare card, all nine Point numbers are shown in the circle. Each line with three Point numbers added across sums 15. That just happens to be the "magic number" of chits allotted each day! (And we did that just for fun with mathematics).

The "cut-out" MagicSquare card on the last page of this book can be used at Practice Circle meetings. Copy to heavier paper, fold, and place the fold-over card in front of you so others can see your name. Then as you complete each chapter Point, fill in the Point dot on your MagicSquare card.

When all 9 Point PRACTICES are completed and the 9 dots are filled, you have completed this training course. Congratulations! And keep going.

Appendix D
MagicHand Chits Page

Here's another way to count chits if you don't want to use the hand drawing and magnets.

Check the box for each chit used. To show your success strike (/) through the DAY when you've stayed at or within the allotted 15 chits—12 palms, 3 thumbs. Vegetables are unlimited—they are included only as a reminder.

DAY	Milk&Dairy			Fruit			Carbs			Protein			Oils&Fats			Vegetables		
Chits	1	2	3	1	2	3	1	2	3	1	2	3	1	2	3	Unlimited!		
1																		
2																		
3																		
4																		
5																		
6																		
7																		
8																		
9																		
10																		
11																		
12																		
13																		
14																		
15																		

16															
17															
18															
19															
20															
21															

Start With 21-Days & Keep going for Life!

Here's another way to Count Chits!

Copy this weekly Chit tally to carry with you— or add to your smartphone.

DAY	Milk&Dairy			Fruit			Carbs			Protein			Oils&Fats			Vegetables
Chits	1	2	3	1	2	3	1	2	3	1	2	3	1	2	3	Unlimited!
Mon.																
Tues.																
Wed.																
Thu.																
Fri.																
Sat.																
Sun.																

Appendix E
SEEING FINGERS on your MagicHand

These lists give a good idea of what foods fall into various food group categories. Some foods can be counted under more than one food group. Note that even though some Vegetables are botanically fruits we still count them as a Vegetables here. You will also find other nuances within groups.

MILK & DAIRY PRODUCTS (palm/cupped portion)	If allergic to Milk & Dairy, below are substitutes high in calcium (use Milk chits for these instead)
Buttermilk	*Almonds*
Camembert	*Canned mackerel*
Cheddar, Farmer's cheese	*Canned salmon*
Cottage cheese	*Canned sardines*
Cream cheese/Neufchatel	*Chickpeas (garbanzo beans)*
Hoop cheese/ Feta cheese	*Dried figs*
Ice cream/Ice milk	*Filberts*
Milk: whole, 2%, skim	*Fortified bread*
Parmesan	*Oats, Oatmeal*
Pudding/custard	*Pistachio nuts*
Swiss cheese	*Red or white pinto beans*
Whipped cream	*Sesame seed*
Yogurt, Kefir	Tofu

High Calcium: Unlimited Foods

Beets	Okra
Broccoli	Parsley
Mustard, collard, turnip greens	Spinach, Kale

FRUIT & FRUIT JUICES *(palm/cupped portion)*

Apples	Olives
Apricots	Peaches
Avocado	Pears
Bananas	Persimmons
Berries	Pineapple
Cantaloupe	Plantain
Cherries	Plums
Cranberries	Pomgranate
Dates	Prunes
Figs	Raisins
Fruit pies	Raspberries
Grapefruit	Strawberries
Grapes	Tangerine
Kiwi fruit	
Lemons and limes	
Mandarins	
Mangos	
Melons	
Nectarines	

CARBOHYDRATES & STARCHY VEGETABLES *(palm/cupped portion)*

Bagels	Ice cream cone
Barley	Lentils
Beans: black, kidney, lima, navy, pinto	Millet
Beer	Muffins
Beets, taro	Oatmeal
Biscuits	Pancakes, waffles
Bran	Parsnip
Breads, rolls	Pasta
Buckwheat	Peas
Cakes, jello	Pita
Cereals	Plantain
Chickpeas	Popcorn
Cookies	Potatoes (all), potato chips
Corn, popcorn	Pretzels
Crackers, croutons	Pumpkin, Yams
Croissants	Rice, rice cakes
Danish pastry	Rye
Doughnuts, cupcakes	Stuffing, bread/rice based
Edamame	Tortillas,, tortilla chips
English muffins, crumpets	Wheat
Grits	Winter squash: acorn, butternut

PROTEIN SOURCES *(palm portion)*

Almonds	Nuts, most varieties
Beef	Organ meats
Black beans	Peanuts
Cheese/ Feta cheese	Pecans
Chicken	Pinto beans
Cold cuts	Pistachios
Duck	Pork
Edamame	Pumpkin seeds
Eggs	Sausages/ frankfurters
Filberts	Shellfish: clams, crab, lobster, shrimp, etc.
Fish: flounder, herring, salmon, sardines, tuna, etc.	Soybeans, tempeh
Game	Sunflower seeds
Goose	Tofu
Green peas	Turkey
Kidney beans	Veal
Lamb	Walnuts
Lentils	Wheat germ
Lima beans	Yogurt
Liver	
Lox/Smoked fish	
Macadamia nuts	
Navy beans	

OILS & FATS AND CONCENTRATED SUGARS *(thumb measure)*

Barbeque sauce	
Butter/Margarine	
Caramel	
Chocolate fudge	
Chocolates	
Coconut oil	
Gravy (oil-base)	
Hard candy	
Ice cream syrup	
Jams and jellies, preserves	
Mayonnaise	
Molasses, Honey	
Nut and seed butters	
Pancake syrup/ maple syrup	
Peanut butter	
Salad dressing	
Sweet sauces, toppings, etc.	
Vegetable oils	

VEGETABLES & HERBS *(unlimited)*

Artichokes	Green, red chilies
Arugula	Green, yellow string beans
Asparagus	Herbs, all
Bamboo shoots	Horseradish
Bay leaf	Jicama
Bean sprouts	Kale
Bok choy	Kimchi
Broccoli	Leeks
Brussels Sprouts	Mushrooms (all)
Cabbage (all)	Mustard greens
Carrots, alfalfa sprouts	Okra
Cauliflower	Olives
Celery	Onions
Chard	Parsley
Chayote	Peppers
Cilantro	Pickles
Cucumbers	Radishes
Eggplant	Rhubarb
Endive	Rutabaga
Escarole	Salad greens, lettuce (all)
Fennel	Salsa/Picante
Garlic	Sauerkraut

VEGETABLES & HERBS *(continued)*

Scallions	Tomatoes
Seaweed (all)	Turnips
Shallots	Vegetable juices
Snap peas, snow peas	Water chestnuts
Spices	Watercress
Spinach	Zucchini
Squash: summer, spaghetti	
Sun chokes	

& Free to use:

baking powder, baking soda	lemon juice, vinegar
chili powder, Worstershire	salt, pepper,
cocoa (unsweetened)	soy sauce, teriyaki
coffee, tea	water, mineral water
flavorings, vanilla	yeast
ketchup, mustard	

Anything missing? Feel free to add to these lists.

Practice Circle Events!

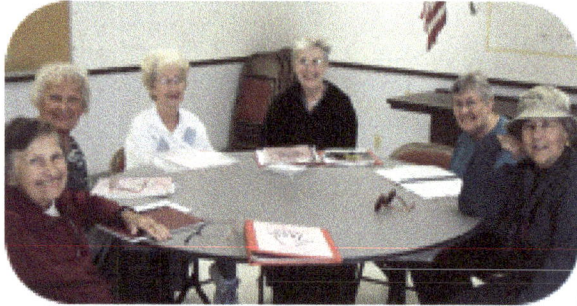

Practice Circle in action! With leader Marilyn Goettsch

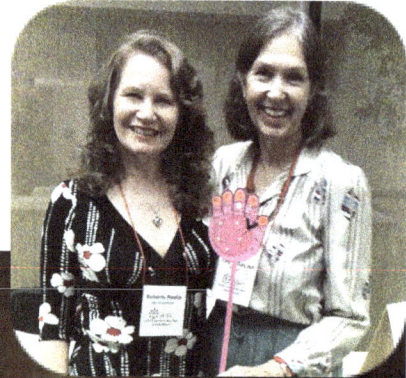

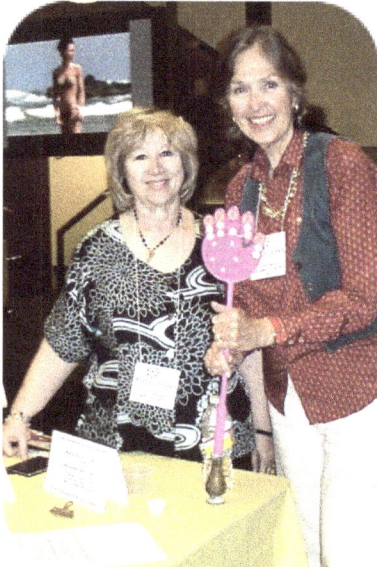

Inviting new members with leader Sandra Kaminsky

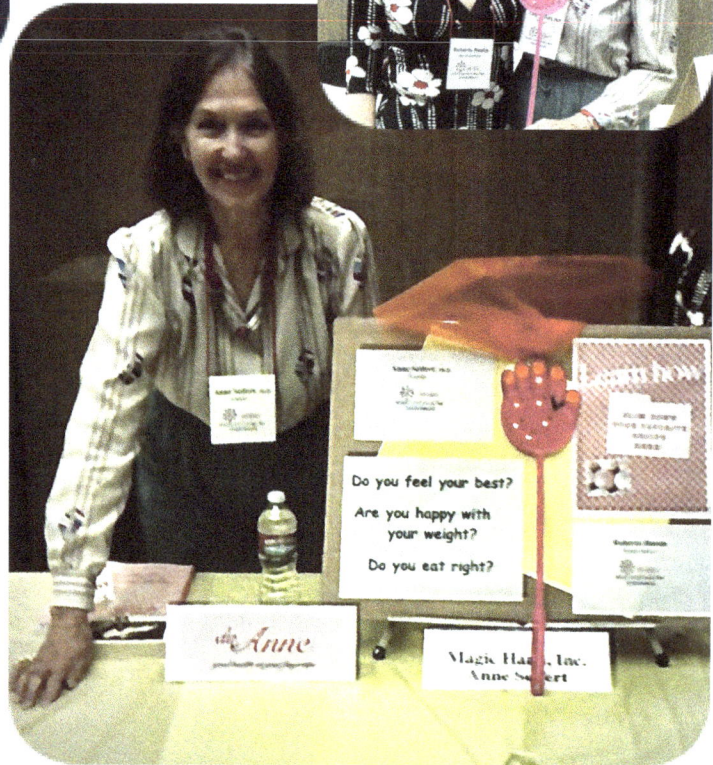

Dr. Anne speaking at Hollywood Screen Actor's Guild Health Fair working with actress Roberta Bassin

Here's the MagicSquare!

Cut and fold, or copy. Fill in the circles as you complete each Practice Point.

Your name here>>>>>

9 lifetime

_____

for:

THE
MAGIC SQUARE

Fold here>>>>>>

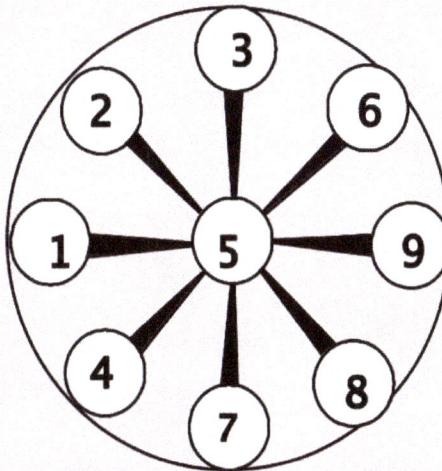

www.ingramcontent.com/pod-product-compliance
Lightning Source LLC
Chambersburg PA
CBHW081421270326
41931CB00015B/3355

* 9 7 8 0 9 4 3 5 8 4 0 4 1 *